SENSORY SUPPORT SERIES

BEFORE THE BRAVE BITE

Empowering Your Sensory Sensitive Child to Explore New Foods

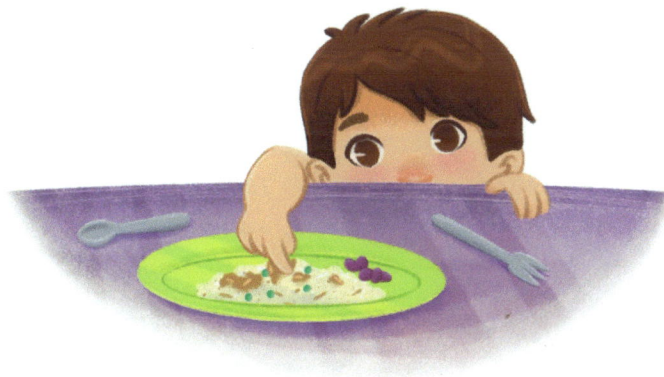

Written by
Madeha Ayub

Illustrated by
Maira Qaisar

GLOBAL BOOKSHELVES
INTERNATIONAL, LLC

Before the Brave Bite: Empowering Your Sensory Sensitive Child to Explore New Foods
Sensory Support Series

Author: Madeha Ayub
Illustrator: Maira Qaisar
Editor: Leila Boukarim
Compositor: Khizra Saeed
Editorial Director: Janan Sarwar

Published by Global Bookshelves International, LLC
Louisville, KY 40241
www.GlobalBookshelves.com

To comment on this book, email globalbookshelves@gmail.com.

Notice
The author and the publisher have made every effort to ensure the accuracy and completeness of the information presented in this book. This book is not intended to serve as medical advice or replace Occupational Therapy (OT) services. Please speak with your child's pediatrician for any health concerns you may have regarding their nutrition. You can also ask if OT services are right for your child in addressing their unique sensory needs.

First Edition
Printed in the United States of America.
ISBN: 978-1-957242-22-4 (Paperback), 978-1-957242-23-1 (Hardback)
Library of Congress Control Number: 2024920472

Dedication

To my husband, Asim, who has always supported my growth as a professional as well as an individual.

And to Sydney and Darwin, who have taken many brave bites since I've met them.

If you ask about my favorite foods
And all the things I love to eat,
It won't take long to tell you that
My list is short, my list is sweet.

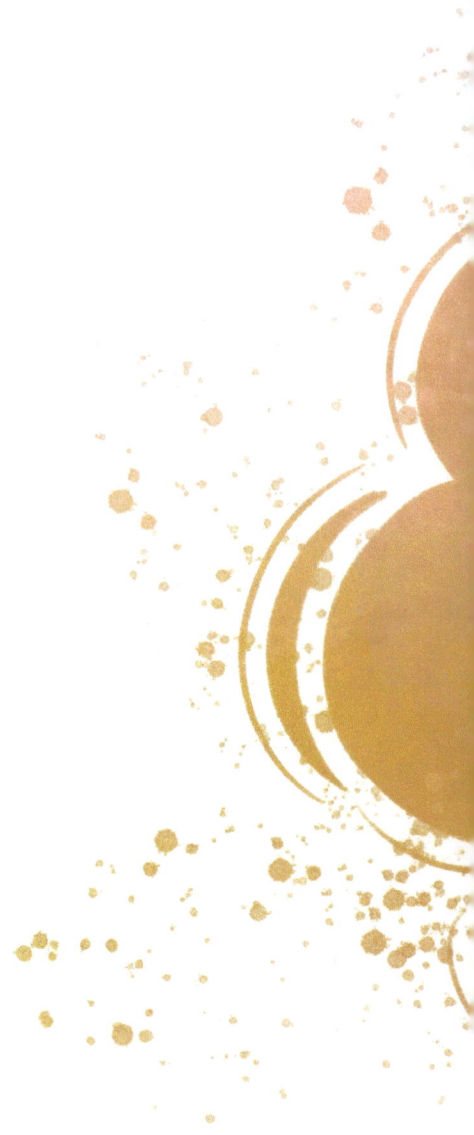

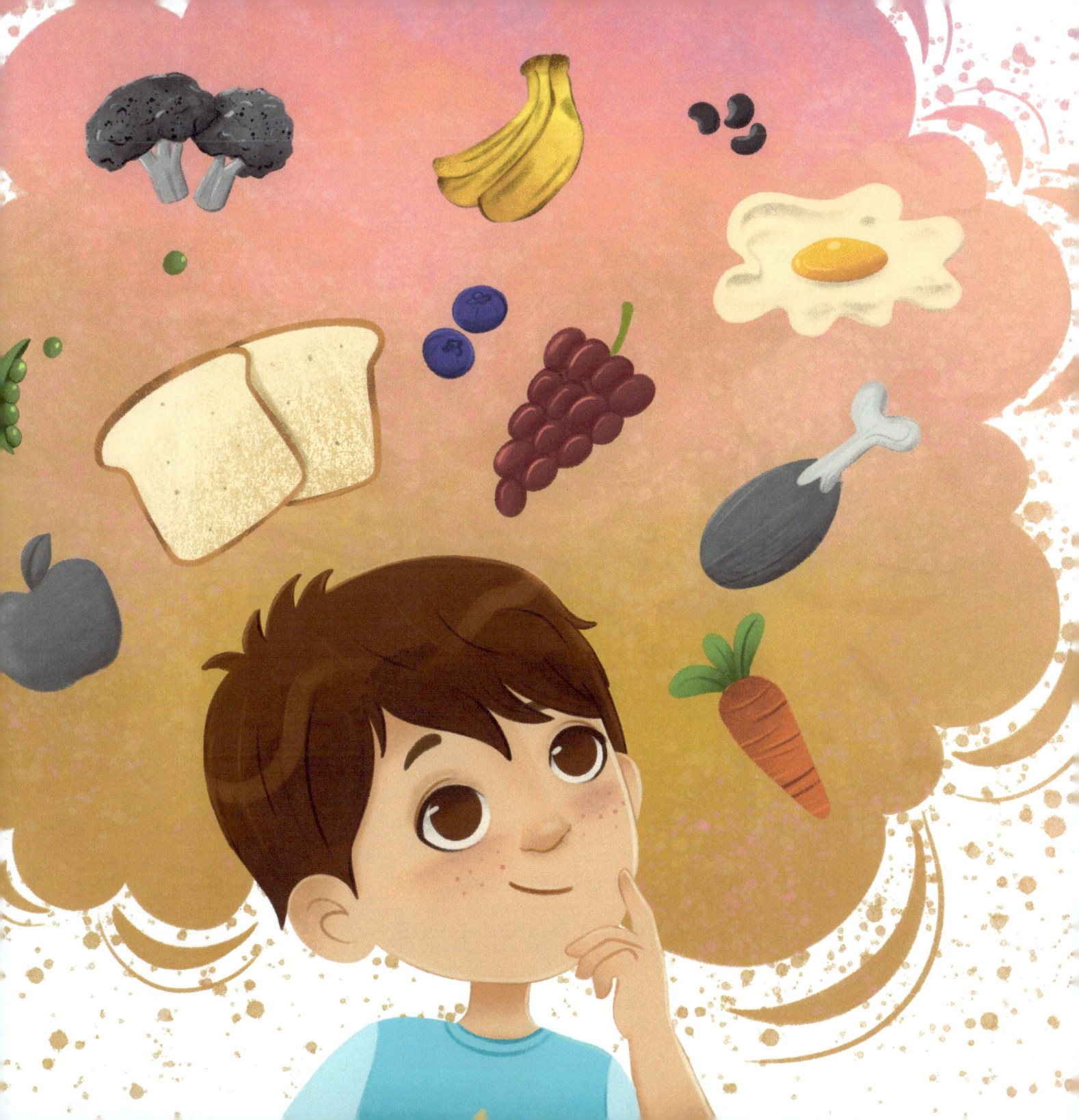

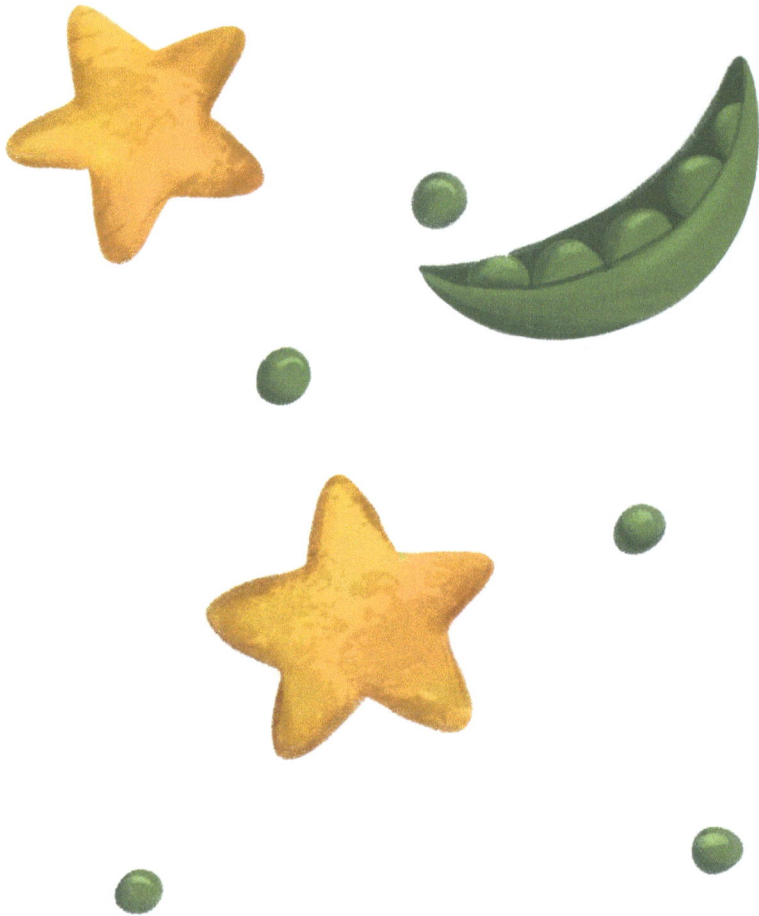

I love my star-shaped chicken nuggets,
A bowl of pasta with cream cheese.
Don't forget my purple grapes,
Or Mom's white rice with green peas.

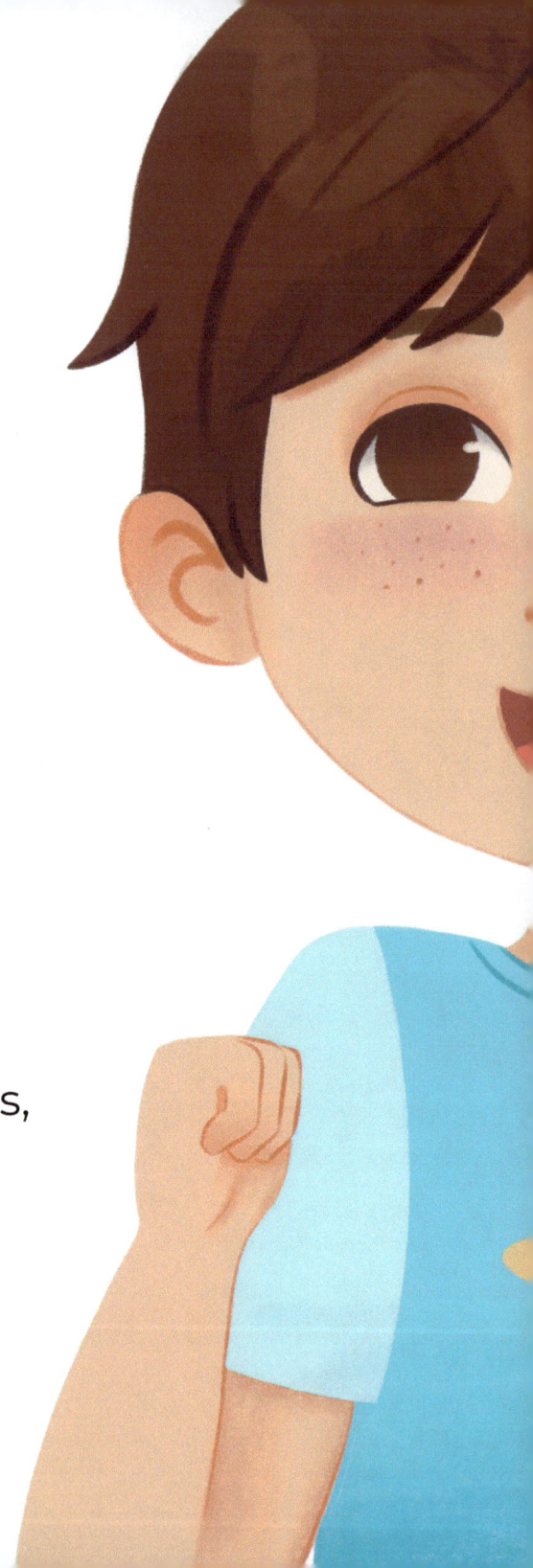

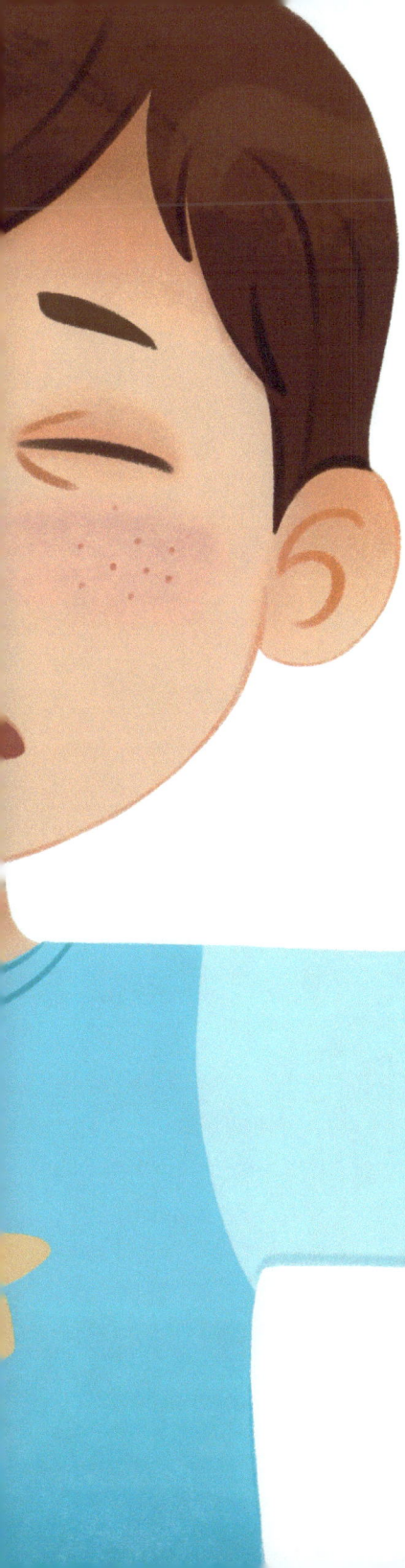

I'll eat this food every day.
My meals are fixed in my routine.
Don't switch peas for lima beans,
Or swap the purple grapes for green.

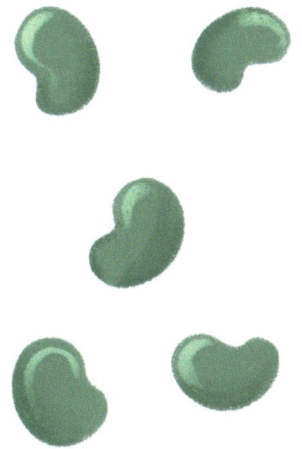

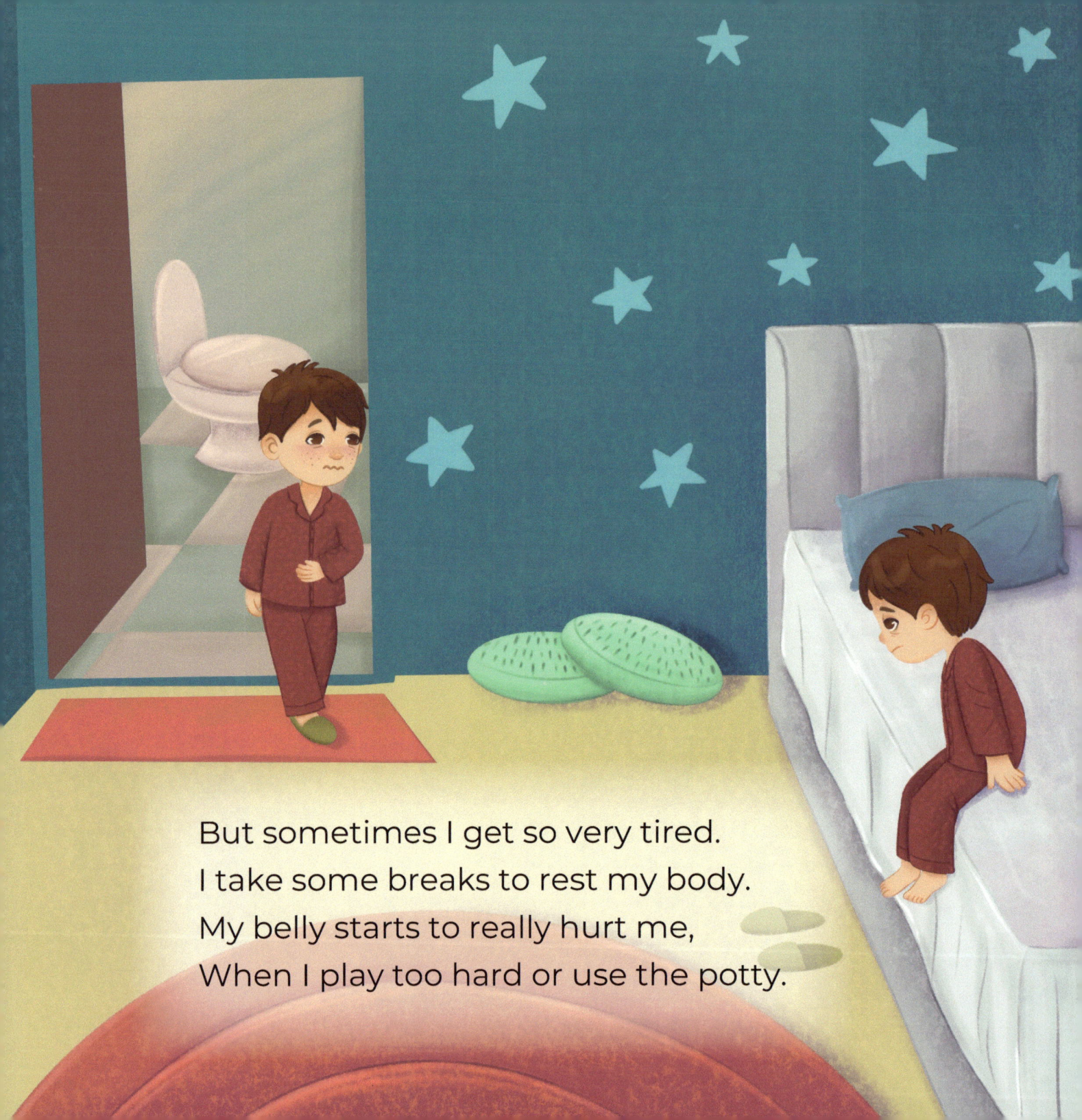

But sometimes I get so very tired.
I take some breaks to rest my body.
My belly starts to really hurt me,
When I play too hard or use the potty.

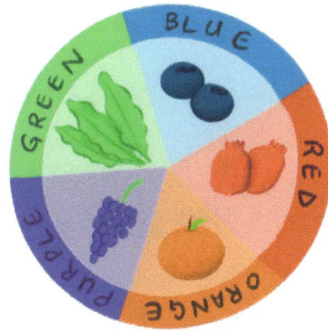

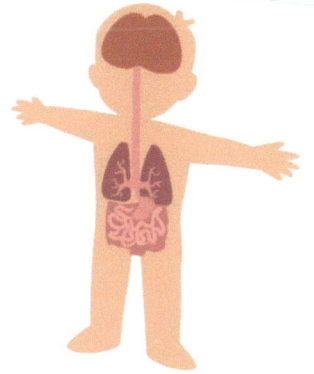

The doctor says that this can happen
When I eat the same food every day.
"Let's add more color to your plate,
So you don't get tired when you play."

The colors in our fruits and veggies
All play a special part.
Green veggies help me not get sick.
Red fruits are healthy for my heart.

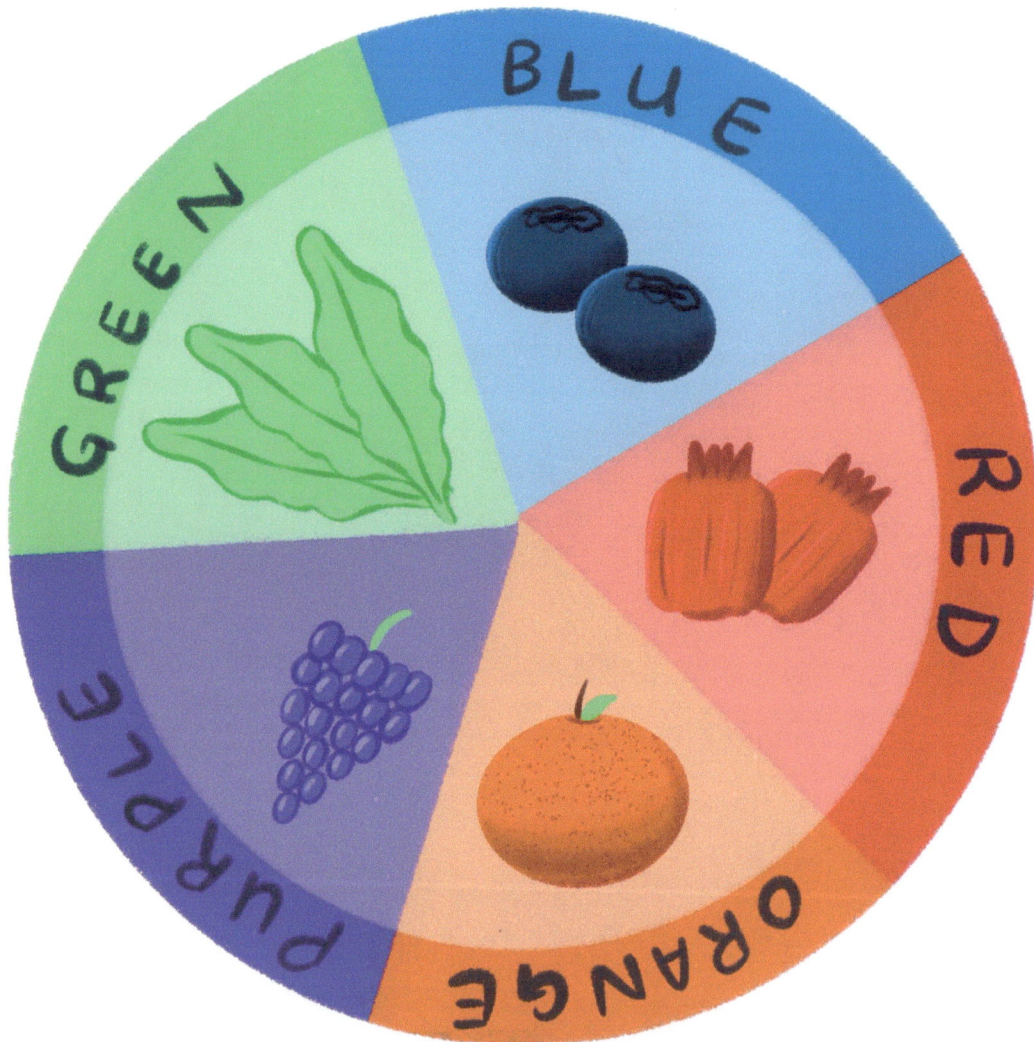

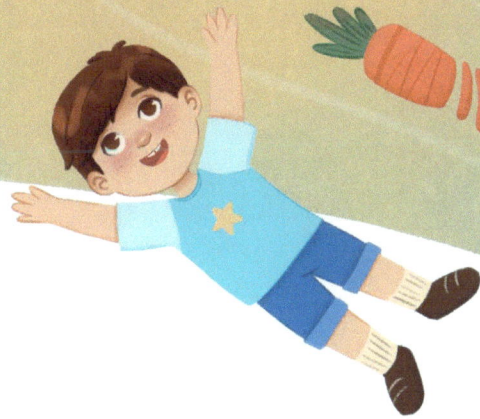

Fruits and veggies aren't as scary
When mixed in rice or stirred in soup.
There are dried fruits, canned fruits, frozen, too—
Great in a smoothie or ice cream scoop.

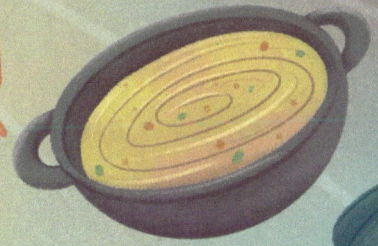

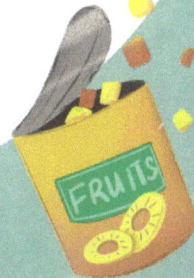

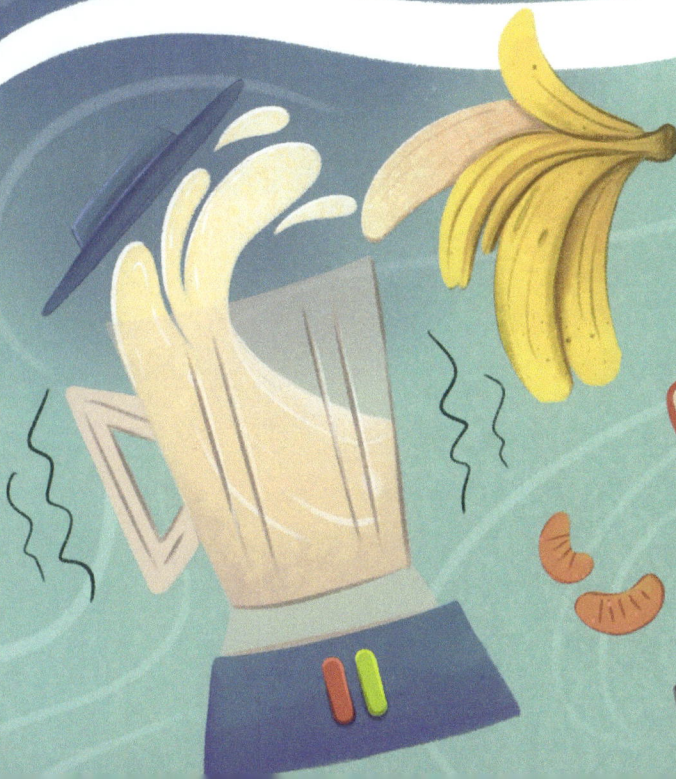

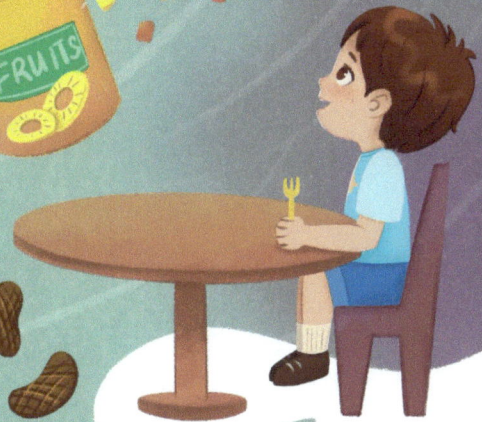

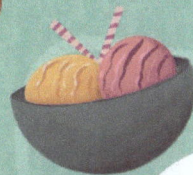

But my brain screams, "No! Don't try this food!
You might get sick, you might throw up!"
My lips are sealed. My mouth stays shut.
My tongue gets scared and then curls up.

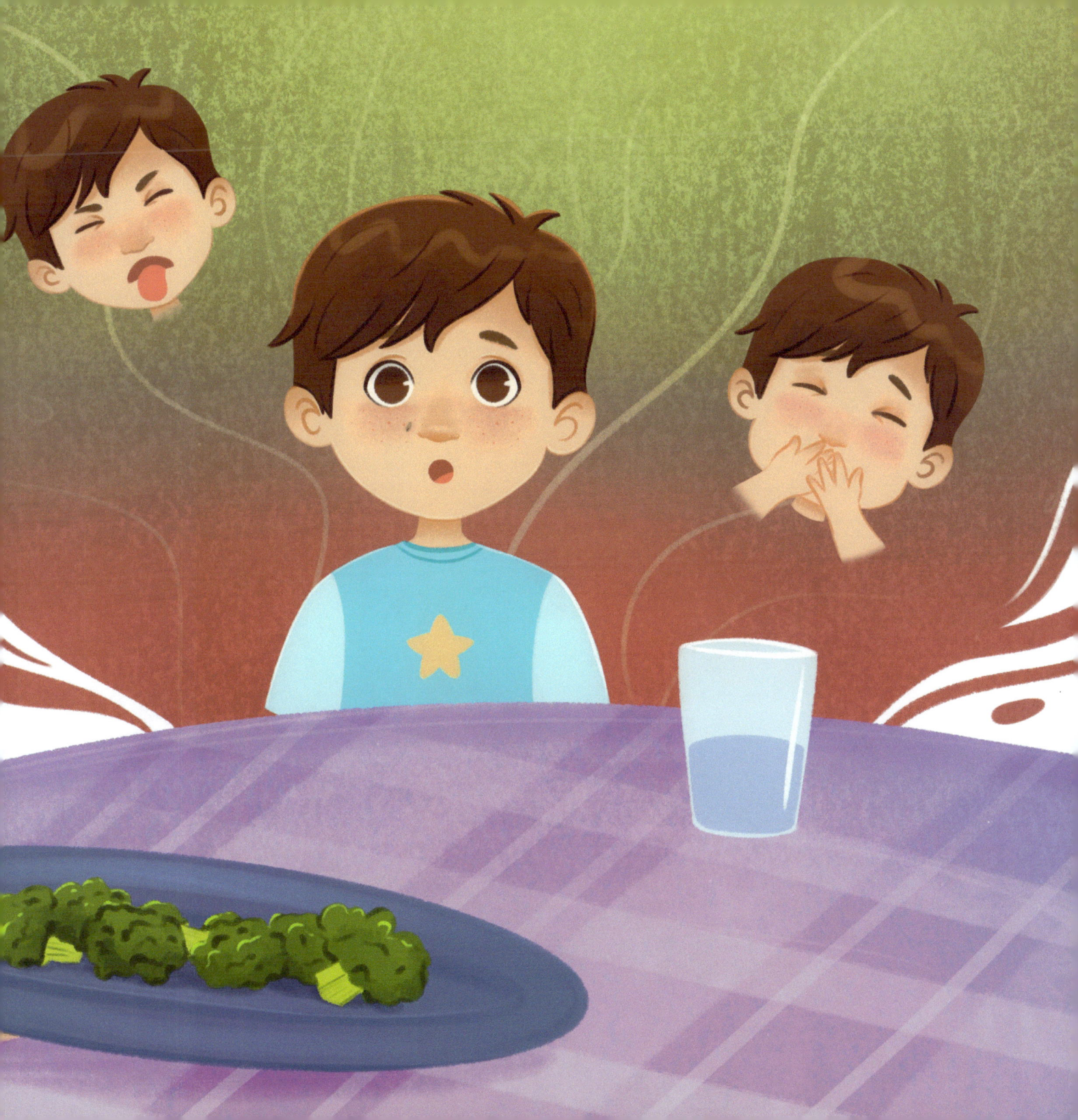

But there are ways for me to try new food,
Or foods I used to like before.
I take small steps; I can't be forced.
I have control to say, "No more."

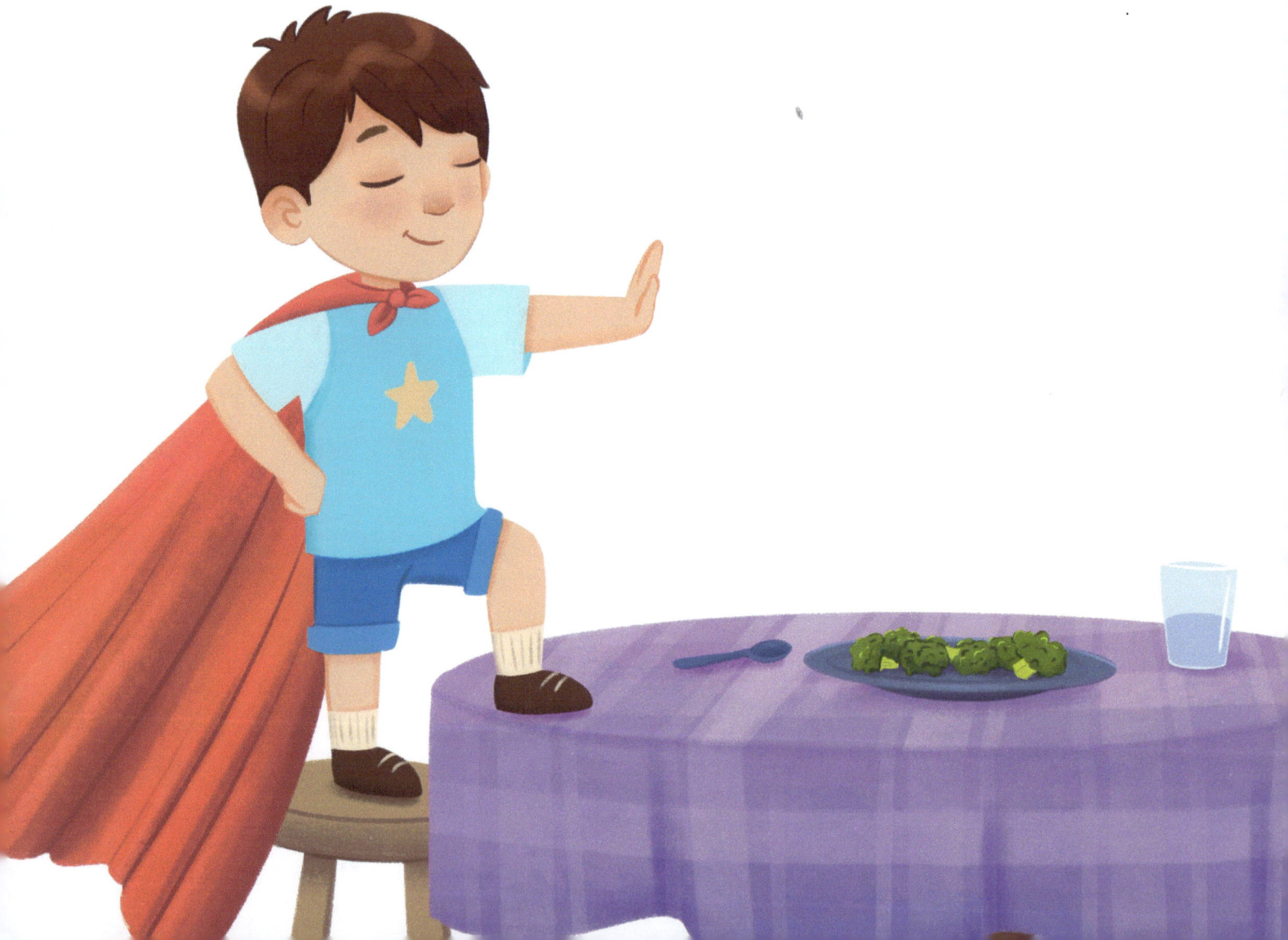

I can start with foods that **feel** the same
As the ones I eat day and night.
Square-shaped nuggets instead of stars,
Or brown fried rice instead of white.

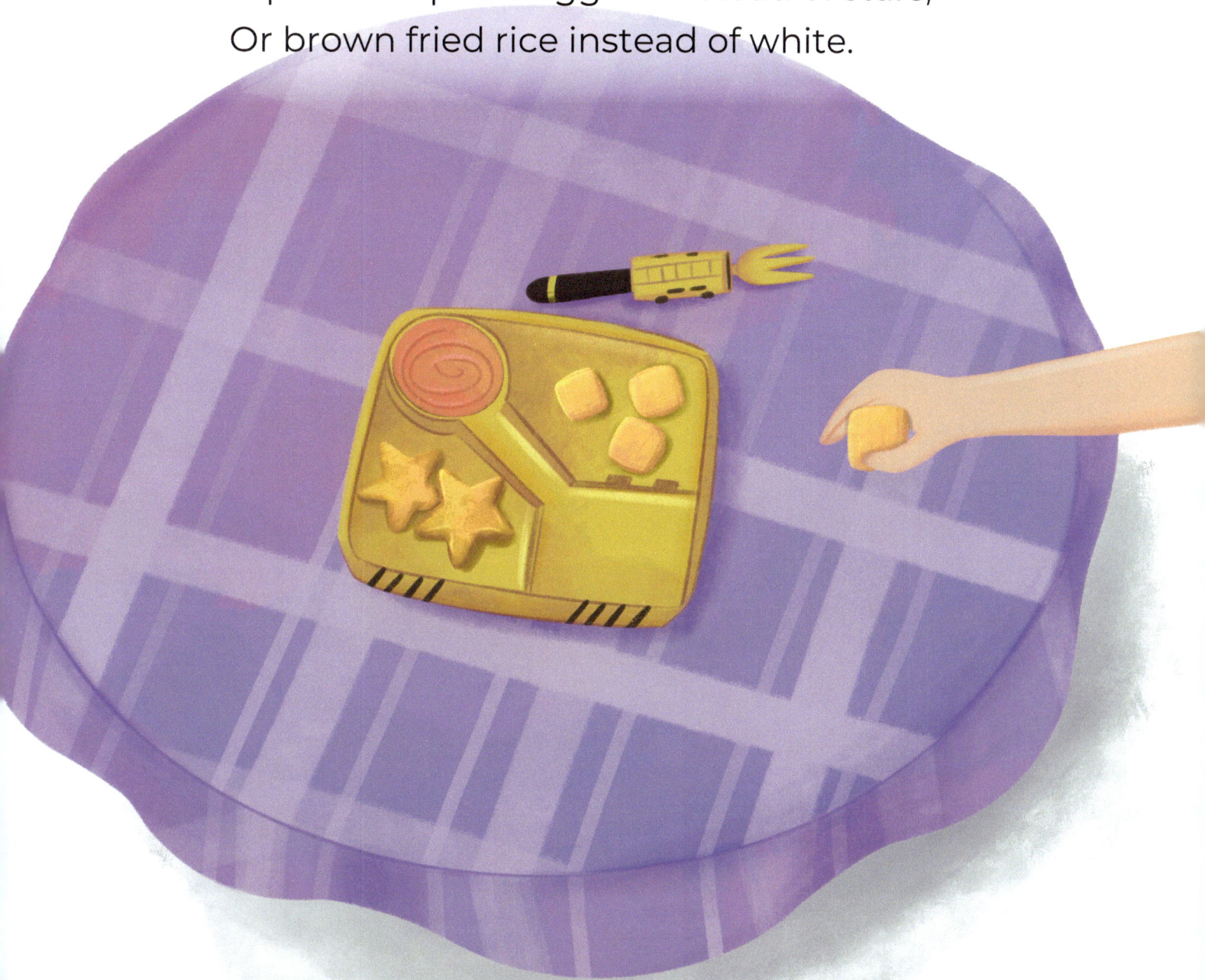

There's fun-shaped pasta that swirls and ties,
On plates and spoons so cool to use.
Mom says we have a secret fruit
That turns my sauce to different blues.

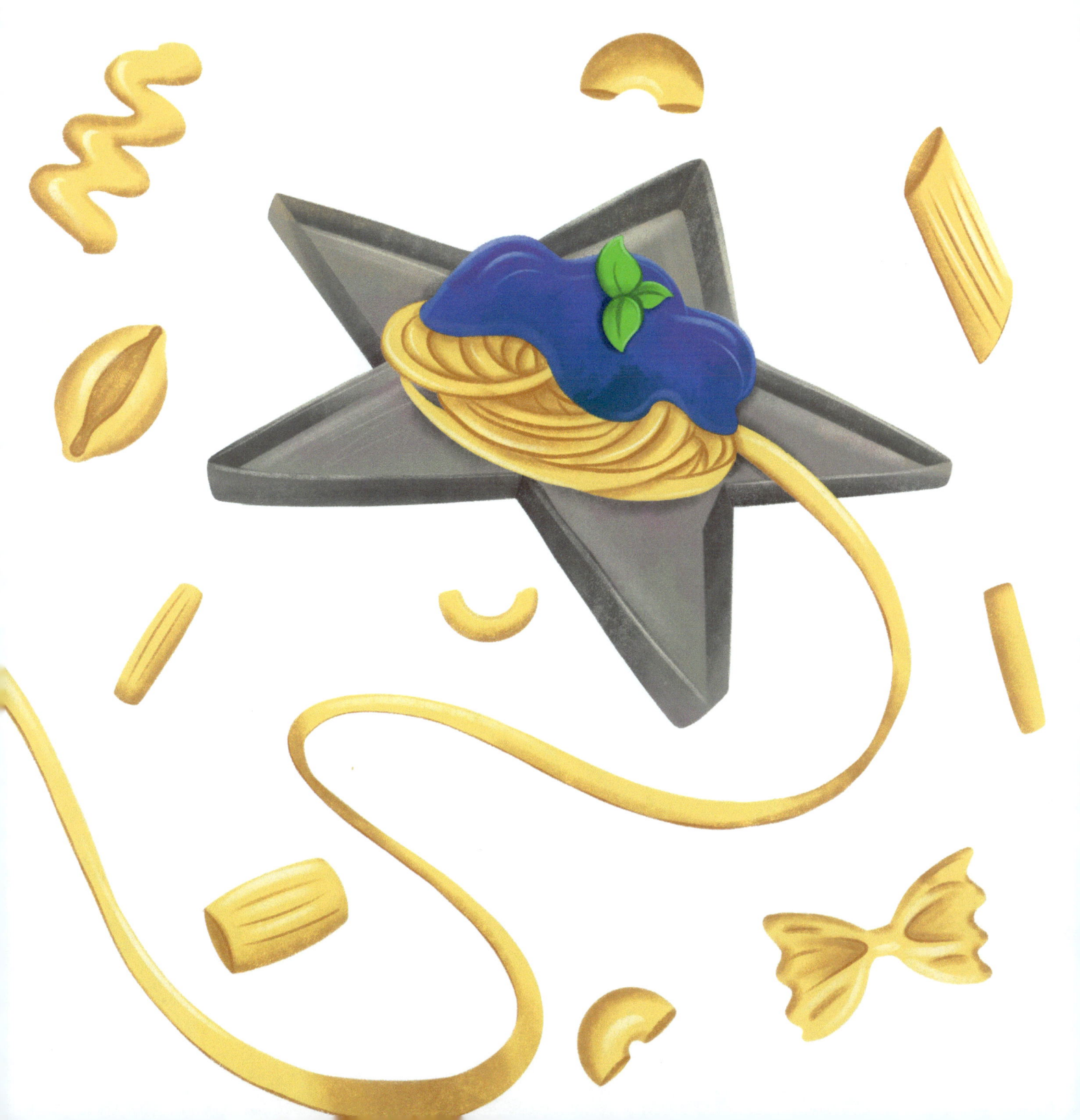

When I decide which food goes first,
To join the table while I eat,
Mom puts it down far from me.
She makes it cold; can't smell the steam.

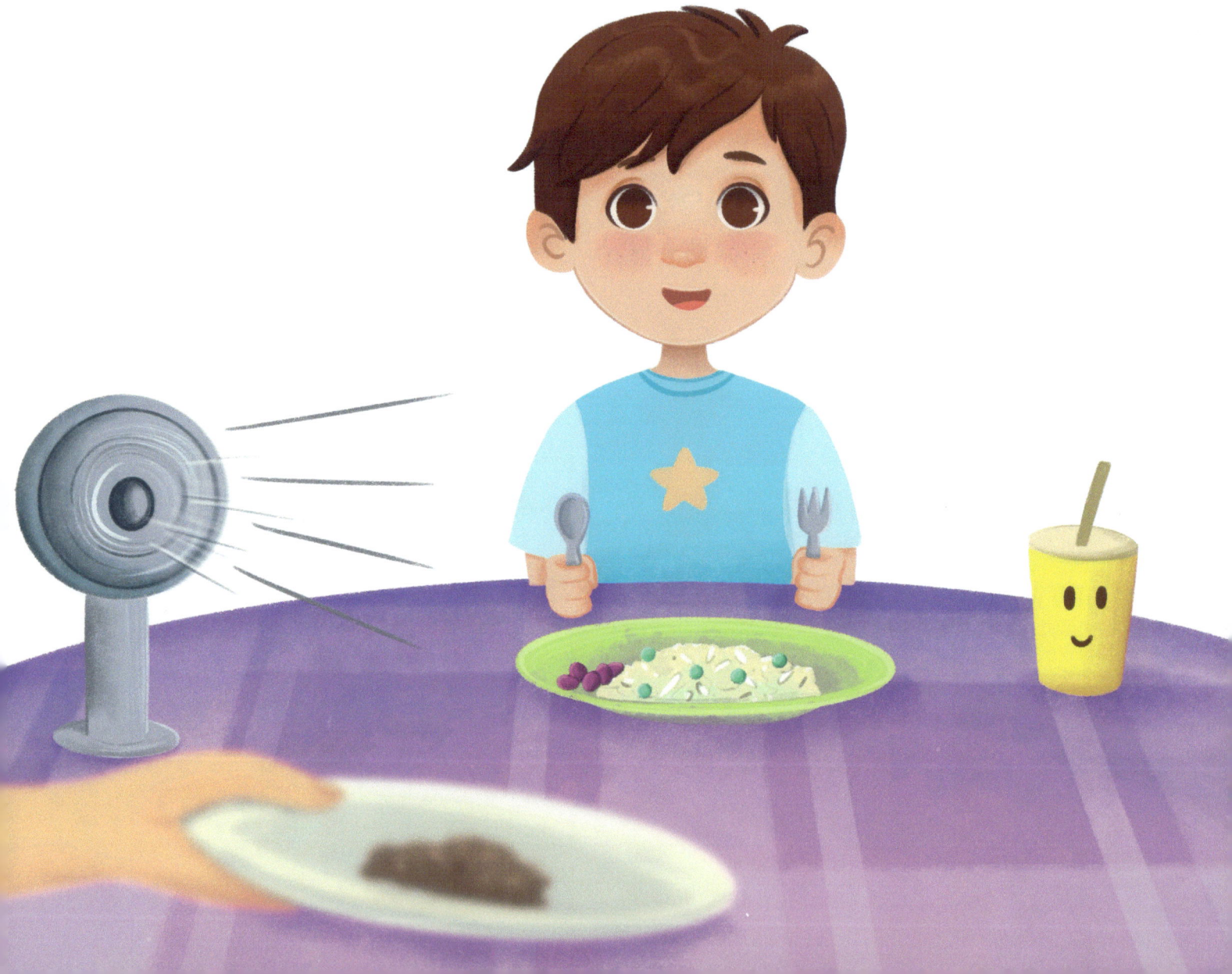

I take small steps and pull the plate.
Level 1, Level 2, Level 3, almost here.
The finish line is next to me.
To win the race, the plate comes near.

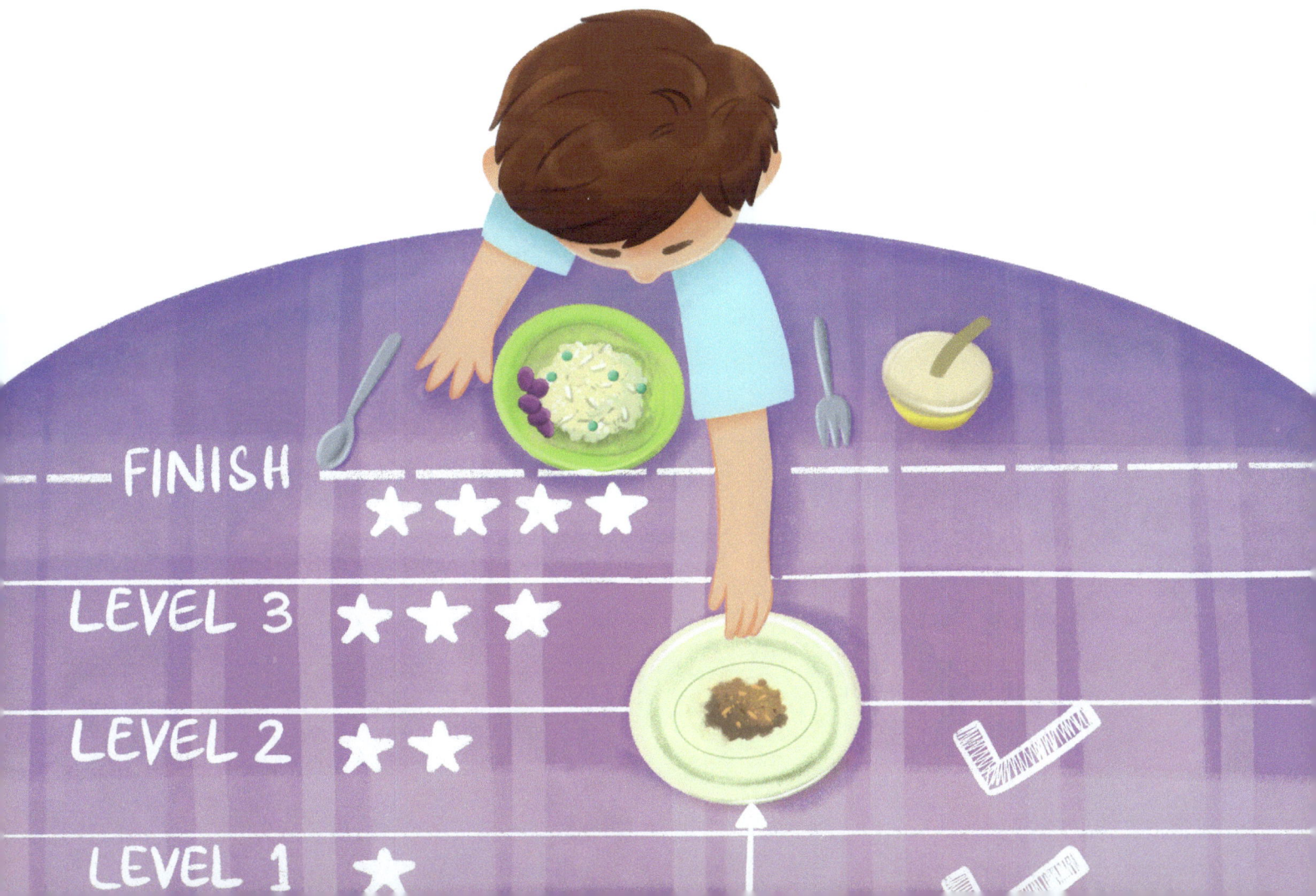

FINISH

LEVEL 3

LEVEL 2

LEVEL 1

Each day, Mom brings the same food back
To the spot it was the meal before.
At times it's hard; it stays in place,
Until I'm ready to pull some more.

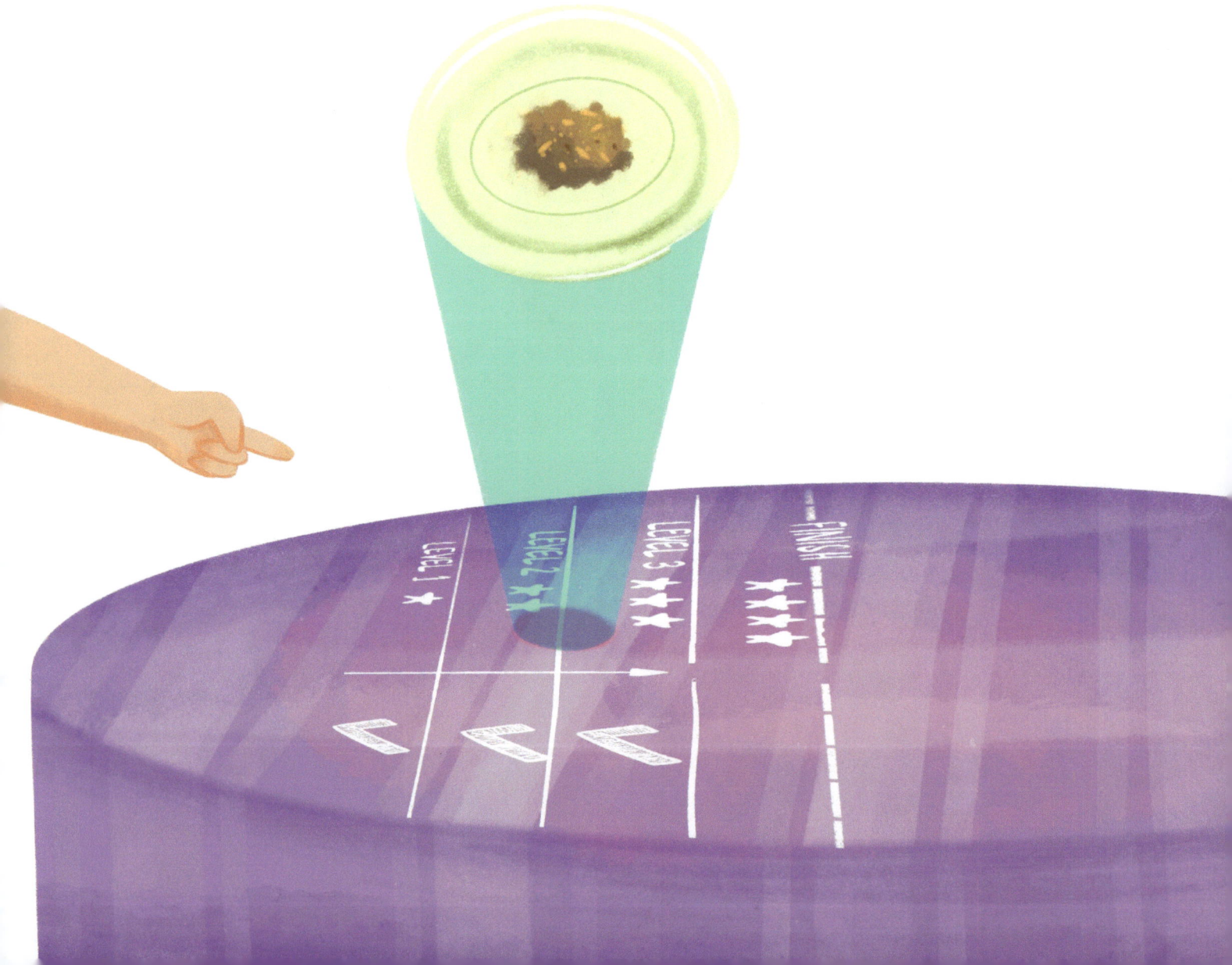

Now the plate comes to a stop.
I'm proud it's here to end the ride.
I don't have to eat the food just yet—
The plates hang out side by side.

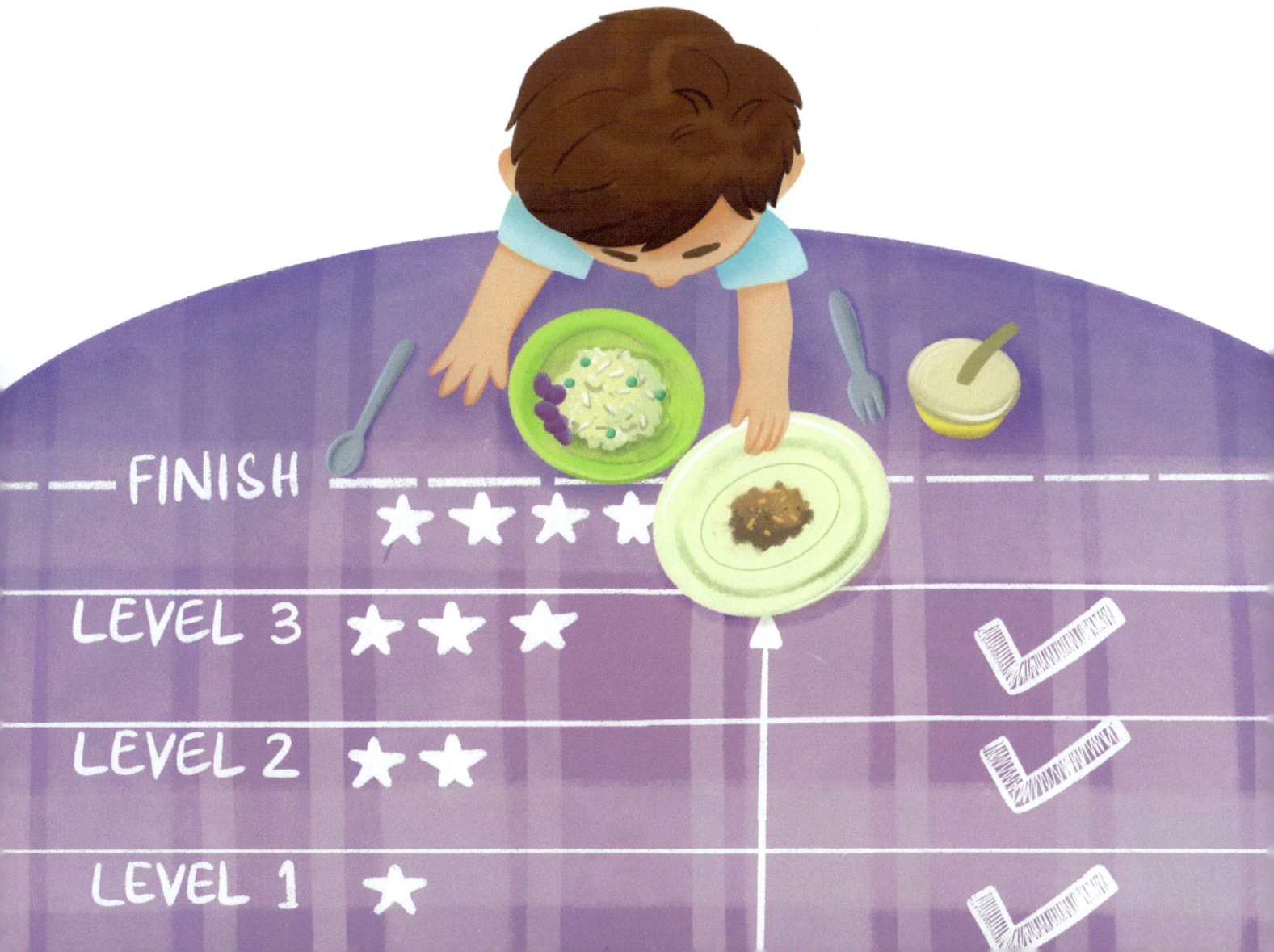

FINISH ★ ★ ★ ★ ★

LEVEL 3 ★ ★ ★

LEVEL 2 ★ ★

LEVEL 1 ★

New food can then hop on my plate—
Away from every rice and pea.
I use a plate with walls so food can't touch,
Or draw magic lines that I can see.

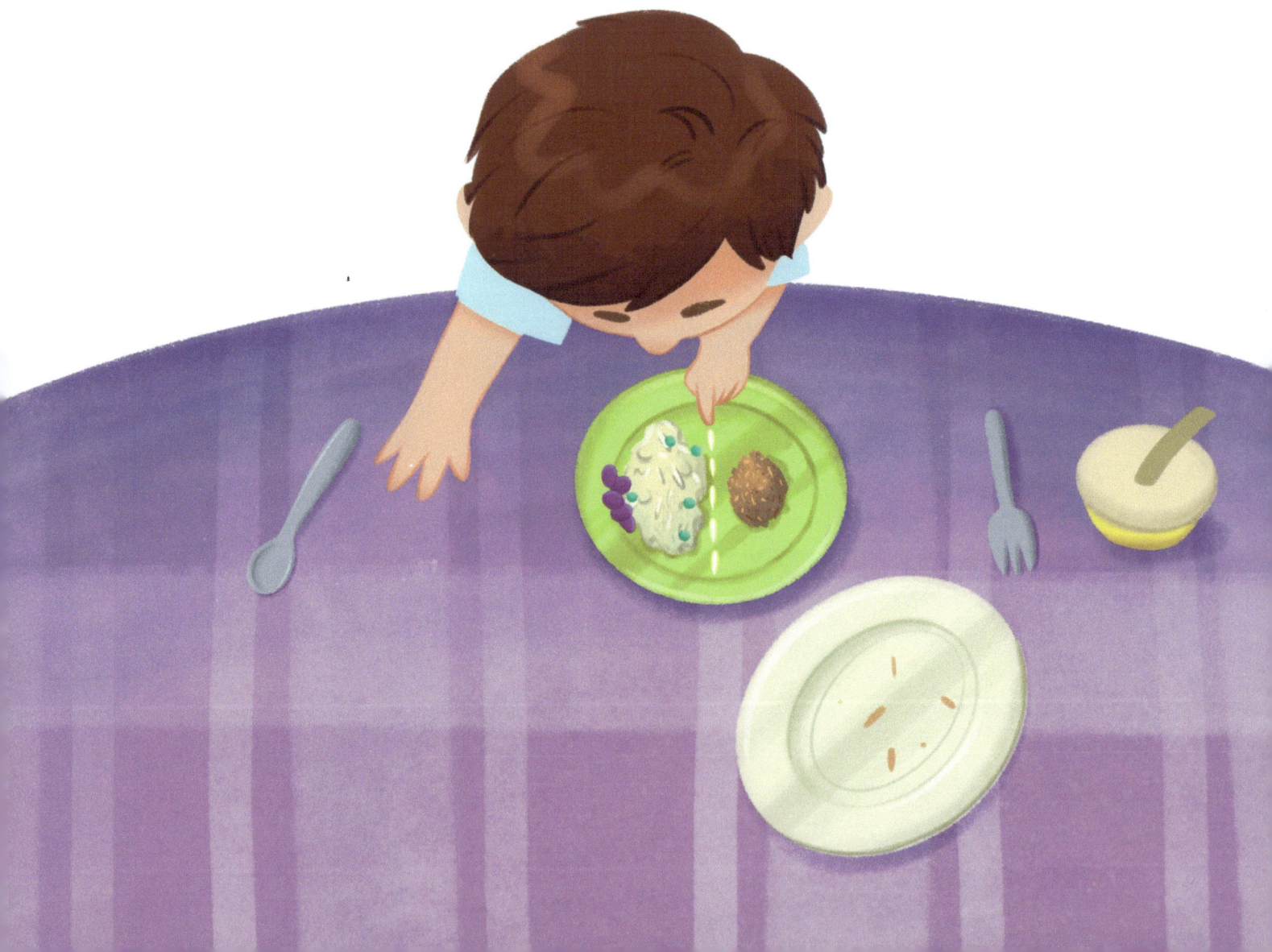

When I am ready, the food can touch,
A tiny bit along one side.
I wonder if Mom's rice tastes good,
Even with bits of brown inside.

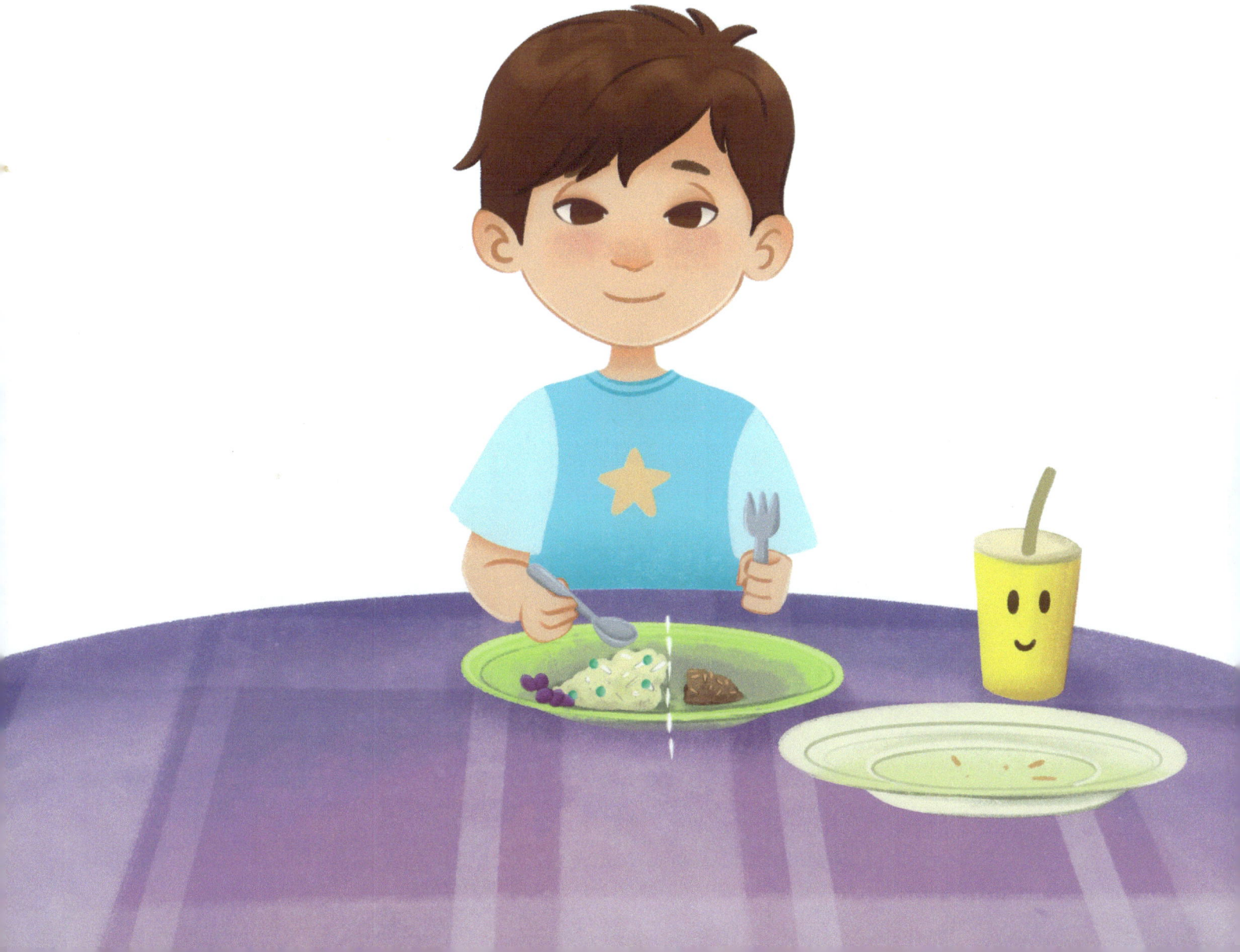

I play with the food and try to smell it.
Poke with my fingers and maybe lick it.

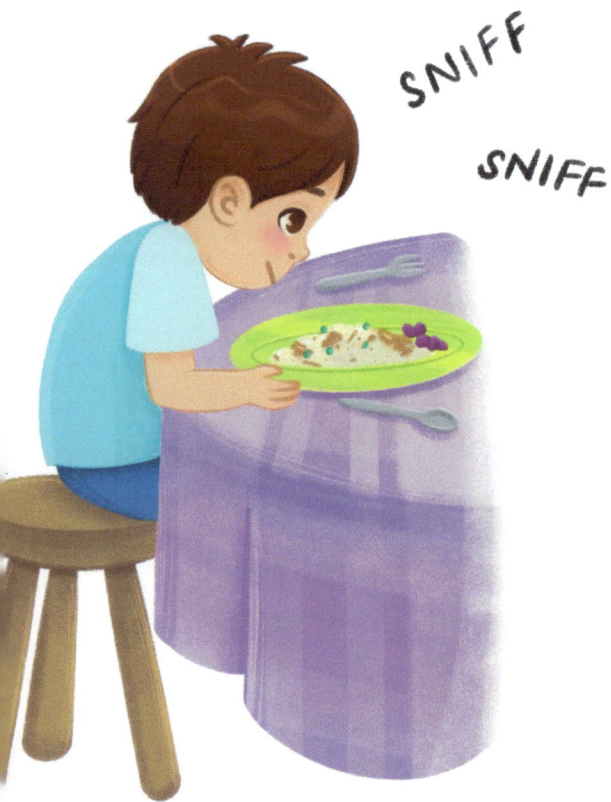

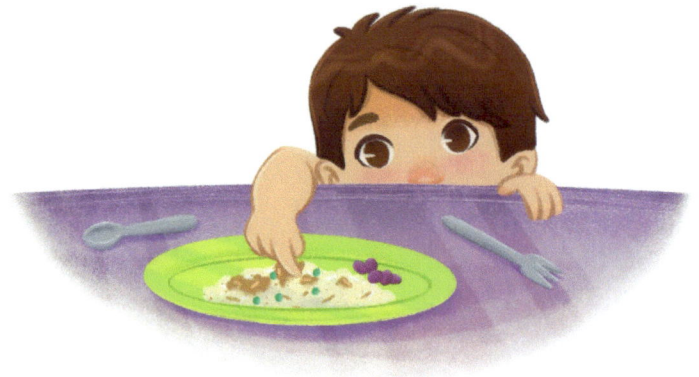

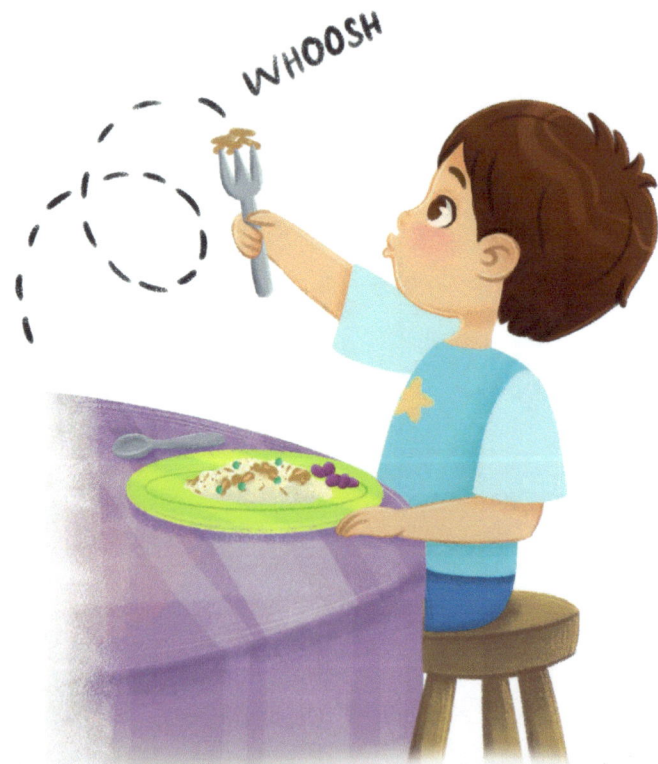

SNIFF

SNIFF

WHOOSH

I pretend it's a dragon fighting my grapes,
Till the grapes grow legs and start to kick it.

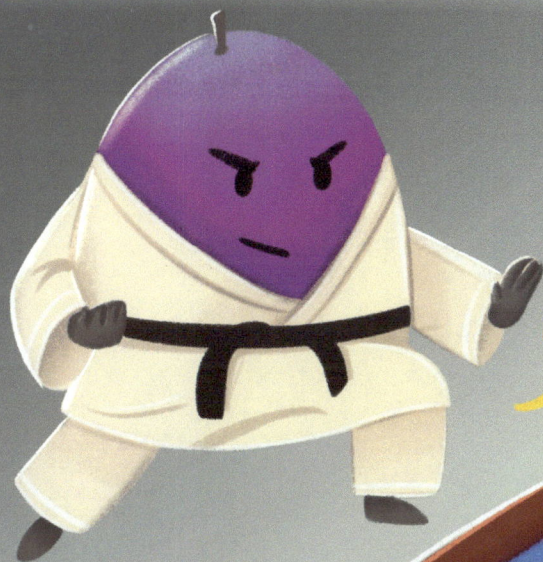

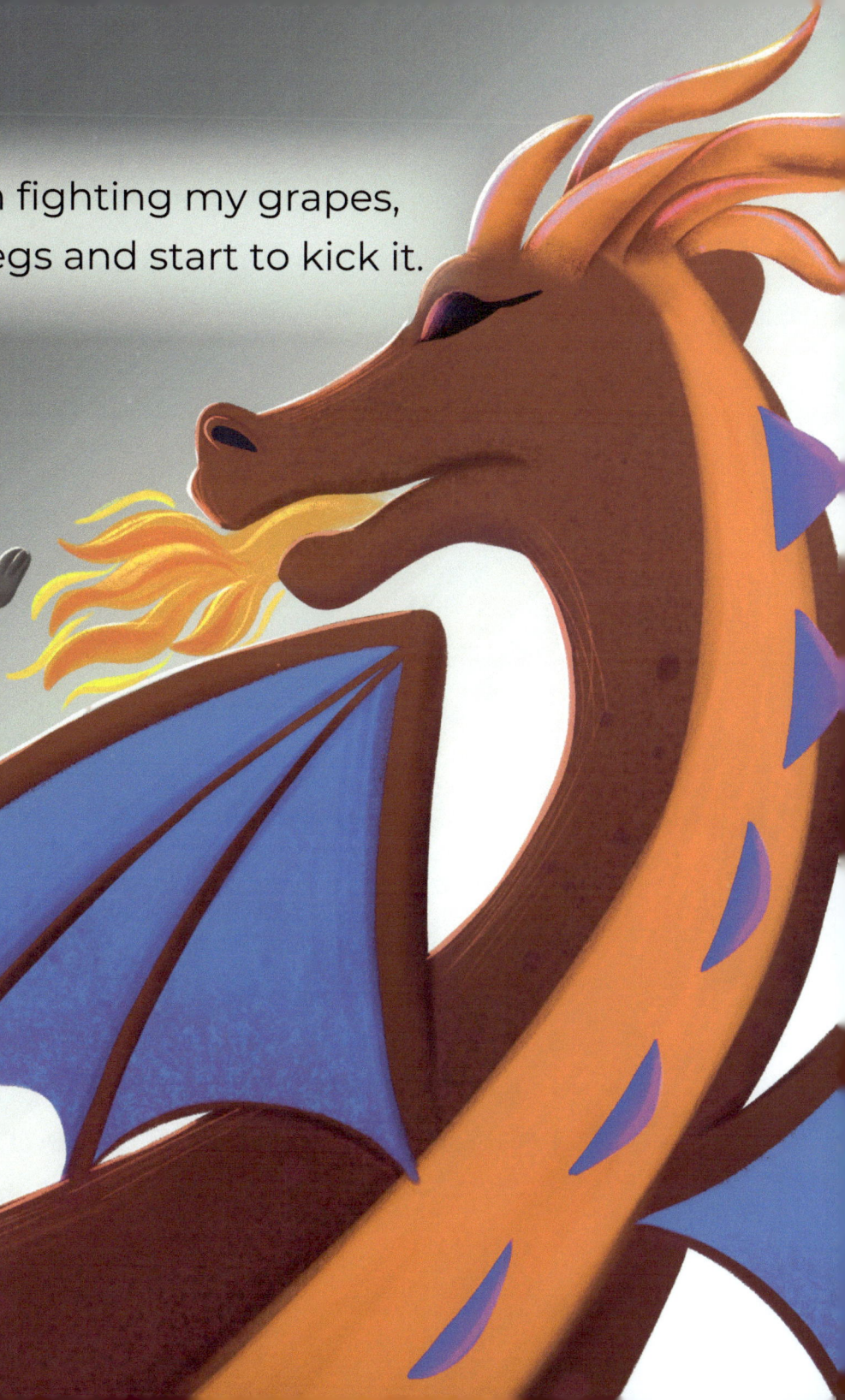

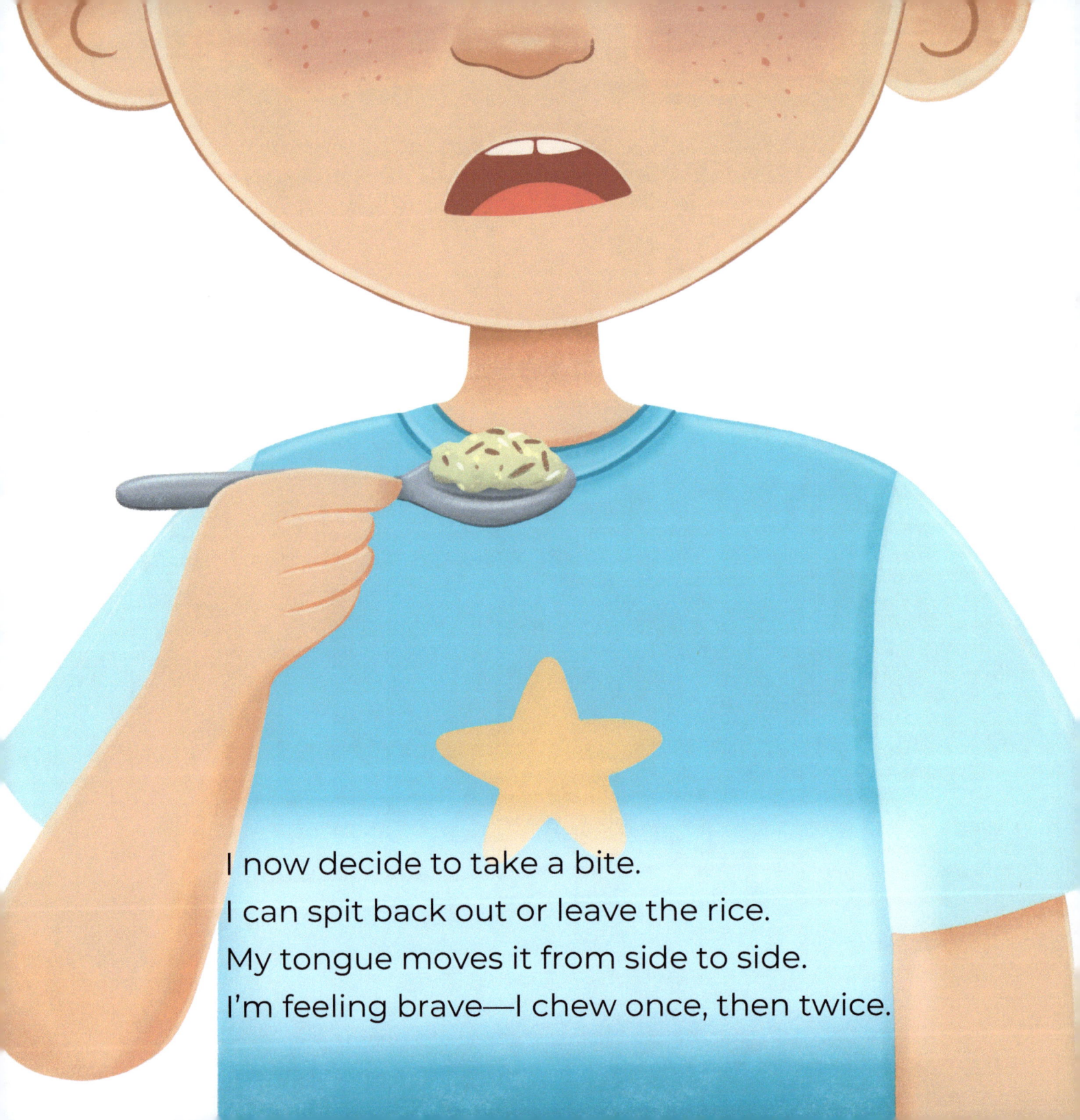

I now decide to take a bite.
I can spit back out or leave the rice.
My tongue moves it from side to side.
I'm feeling brave—I chew once, then twice.

A tiny bite goes down my throat.
I don't want more, and that's all right.
I wait to see if I feel sick.
But, hmm, I don't! I feel all right!

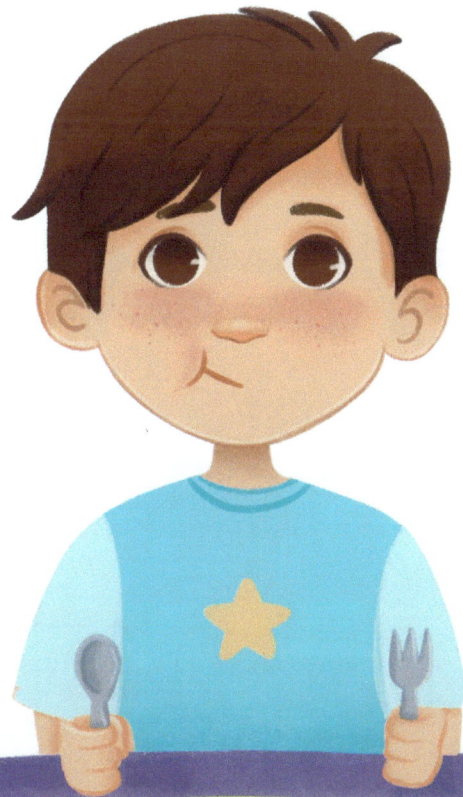

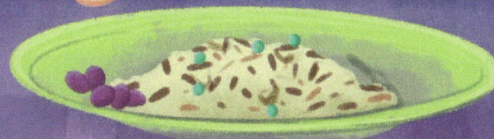

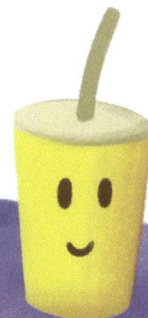

What's more surprising than the bite
Is I may like the food I try.
I'll add it to my list of favorites;
This list will slowly multiply.

I did my best to try new foods,
At a pace that feels most right.
When I am ready to try more things
I won't forget what comes before...

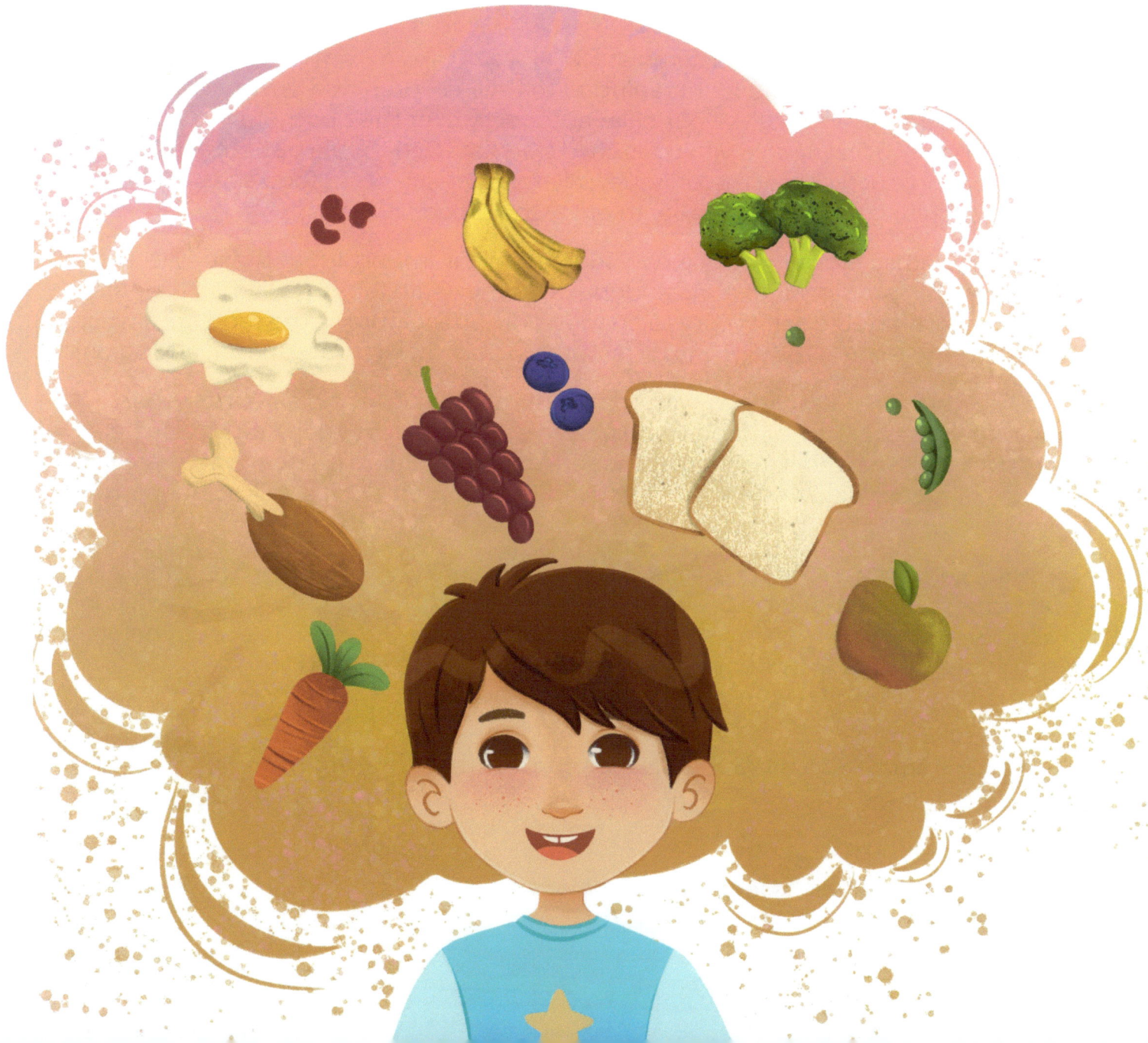

My next brave bite!

A Word to Caregivers

Children with sensory aversion to foods are more than just selective eaters. Their brains will label aversive foods as life-threatening, which can often lead to anxiety, nausea, gagging, and in severe cases, vomiting.

As a pediatric Occupational Therapist (OT), I would like to remind caregivers that new food introductions should be meaningful to their children and enhance their quality of life. It is important to give your child autonomy over their body each step of the way. Be sure to first speak with your child's pediatrician to rule out other reasons for picky eating, such as oral motor issues, allergies, or any other food sensitivities that may be limiting your child's ability to enjoy their food.

Once your child is ready to try a new food item, it is important to begin with food textures that are similar or almost identical to their safe foods (i.e., foods they are already comfortable eating). Try to change only one feature of the food item while keeping the texture the same (e.g., features include color, shape, flavor, and so on).

Having your child simply play with unfamiliar food is a fun and safe method to help them associate new foods with comfort and joy. Pediatric OTs can also help create a personalized sensory diet that ensures your child's sensory needs are met throughout the day, which will better prepare their body to feel calm and ready for mealtime.

Finally, celebrate all the wins! Taking a bite is not the only achievement. Every step in the process, whether it be deciding which food to try first, smelling the item, licking it, or even chewing it before spitting it back out, is applaudable. The steps before the brave bite all help to promote comfort and safety around new foods.

Use the board game at the end of the book to boost motivation!

Visit my website SeedsforSpecialNeeds.com for more resources.

Follow @seedsforspecialneeds
on Instagram!

With love,
Madeha

Use a small toy or a game piece from another board game to move along the phases of new food introduction!

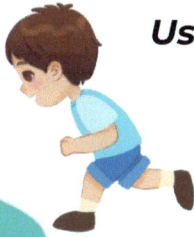

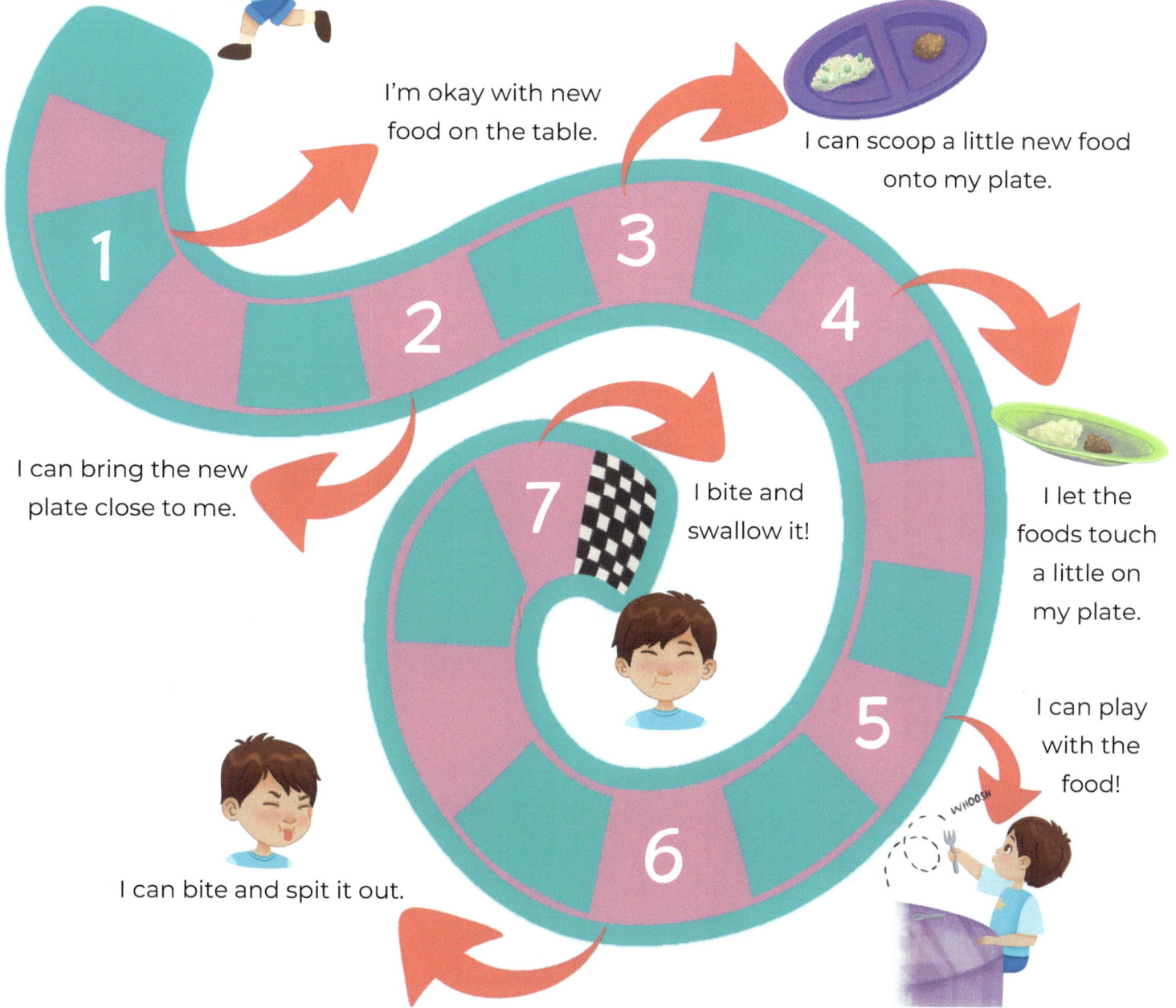

1

I'm okay with new food on the table.

I can scoop a little new food onto my plate.

2

3

4

I can bring the new plate close to me.

I let the foods touch a little on my plate.

7

I bite and swallow it!

5

I can play with the food!

WHOOSH

6

I can bite and spit it out.

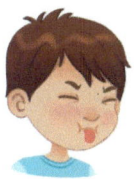

www.ingramcontent.com/pod-product-compliance
Lightning Source LLC
Chambersburg PA
CBHW041105050426
42335CB00046B/128